I0476583

The Snoring Cure

Reclaiming Yourself From Sleep Apnea

By Luke Mattheson

Table of Contents

Introduction

Snoring is Not Only Annoying
Snoring is not just something people do, it is a symptom; snoring is a manifestation of damage that caused by an underlying issue. Because snoring has been wrongly considered a part of many, if not most people's sleeping habits, the damage that causes people to snore has gone unrecognized in most people, this is true even today.

What is The Damage?
Sleep is the recuperative process we must have in order to be healthy and sharp. Snoring is a disturbance that can interrupt our sleep, causing us to wake up from trouble snoring represents in our ability to breathe well, and even from the noise snoring can generate. Snoring is just a problem

the snoring person alone must deal with; this is something that can affect anyone within earshot, especially a partner sleeping in the same bed, or someone sharing the room. Another person snoring can keep a person from getting truly restful sleep; this can be absolute torture for a person who must share a bed or sleeping quarters with someone who snores.

Noise is the least of the problems snoring causes. In its ultimately damaging form, people die, not from snoring, but Sleep Apnea. Snoring is just the audible manifestation of Sleep Apnea, which is the term for when a person involuntarily stops breathing while asleep. It is the Sleep Apnea is that causes a snorer to breath so heavily, not to mention loudly. Sleep Apnea is what causes a person to wake up gasping, or to adjust their sleeping position over and over throughout the night. A lack of deep rest has a cumulative degenerative effect on a person, affecting their mood, temperament, and ability to focus, concentrate and be a productive individual.

How Bad Can It Be?

Snoring is often depicted as being cute, or humorous in the sense of how ridiculous a persons snoring can be, but let see how funny you think it would be if you were in that position. If you have never had to sleep with a person who snores, consider this a blessing in your life; now let us compare the often bombastic nature of a persons snore. The following examples should give you an idea of what so many people must endure when trying to get a good nights rest; each of these items registers at least the number of decibels as the average person who snores:

- A gas powered lawn mower in use
- A shop vacuum in use
- A motorcycle in use
- A low flying airliner
- A chainsaw in use
- All of your kitchen appliances running at the same time

Snoring is a Constant Issue

The point to remember about these examples is that you are subject to them for the entire time you are trying to get rest; deep, uninterrupted, quality sleep. This is not blowing things out of proportion, talk to anyone has slept with someone who snores what it is like and you will get an earful, so be prepared to listen. Snoring is not like the hiccups, it does not go away as suddenly as it appeared, snoring will be a persistent issue until something is done about it, or the snorer dies in their sleep.

Why Are You Reading This?

If you are reading this chances are either you, the person you spend your nights with or someone you care about snores and it is driving one of you, if not both of you absolutely crazy. Losing sleep is hugely detrimental. And it can make you feel a little crazy when you are faced with a wall of noise that stands between you and the sleep you so need and deserve, every night.

You are reading this because you are looking for a solution. You don't want to keep snoring, or you definitely want your sleeping partner to stop snoring. Don't get the impression that this is a brochure for snore resolving surgery, it is not. This book provides some very simple answers and solutions that can make all the difference in the world; these solutions have not only eradicated snoring, but are actually life savers. These non surgical solutions can get back the sleep you need as someone who snores, or as a person who sleeps with someone who snores; either way the will be more sound sleep to go around.

Before proceeding, we need to take the time to understand snoring at its most basic level; the physical components involved in the process.

Once we understand how snoring works we can delve deeper into looking at it's problematic nature. At this point we will study the harmful process of snoring, the negative effects it has and what it represents in the human body.

Once we understand what snoring is and what it can mean, we can then proceed into how to remedy the snoring dilemma. When it comes to solutions to biological processes, understanding the surgical procedures first; in order to understand how and why this option to snore resolution is a risky decision and in many cases does not help at all. By the end of all this reading, you perception of snoring will be drastically changed; snoring will not be funny or acceptable for you or anyone you care about.

Chapter One: Understanding Snoring

Snoring is understood to be any kind of resonant sound that emanates from breathing while sleeping. The crux of the snore is where the mouth and nasal passages meet; this is the point where breathing during sleep causes vibration; otherwise known as snoring. This vibration is due to constricted breathing passages. As tight breathing passages are responsible for snoring, it should also be understood that the more pinched these passages are, the louder and more disruptive the snoring will be.

The reason snoring only occurs while slumbering is because the body is in a prone position in a relaxed state. The airway consists of tissues that operate in a similar method to muscles. When a person sleeps, these tissues become somewhat flaccid; so when lying down this tissue literally blocks the breathing passage causing the sleeper to breath with difficulty, resulting in more forceful breathing which then equates to snoring.

What Factors into How Loud a Person Snores?
Every person is unique in their composition and physical make up. This affects why some people snore at a very loud volume. Included as part of snoring the tone and pitch; basically

we all have the same parts yet we all have our own uniquely identifiable voice, this is true for snoring as well.

How loud an individual may snore depends on the various factors involved in the process. Because there is basically a flap of tissue closing off the airway we need to breathe, breathing becomes more labored and aggressive to supply our lungs, body and brain with oxygen; snoring is an audible sign that the body is fighting for air. This is an issue that can affect just about anyone, even babies.

The smaller the passages involved with breathing are during sleep, the more forceful the body will become in an effort to get the air it needs, thusly the tissue blocking the airway will vibrate in proportion to the force needed to get the vital oxygen our body is being

deprived of. This is how a snore
becomes so loud.

Men Snore the Most
Generally speaking, men do most of
the snoring that goes on in the world.
This has to do again, with the physical
composition of the male body; in this
case, the neck, which is typically
thicker. Because the male neck is more
often fleshier in nature, there is more
tissue substance found within.
Obviously, the more tissue there is in
the neck and surrounding the
breathing passages, the greater the
likelihood of bombastic snoring.

Women have a natural defense to
snoring in the form of Progesterone.
Granted, there are woman who snore
just a loud and violently as men, and
even more so in some cases, but it is
simply not as common as it is with
males. Progesterone is used as a form

of therapy for men who suffer from snoring.

Snoring: Causes and Amplifiers

As we have already discussed, snoring is a symptom of something else. This symptom manifests in the form of a sound that comes from the inability to breathe easily during sleep. So what causes this trouble? The tissues involved with breathing are not the sole culprit for this bothersome problem. These factors are not gender specific; these are issues that affect men and women, although there are roughly twice as many male snorers as there are females who snore. Snoring factors have to do with our health and our lifestyle; these factors come in many combinations and include the following:

• Allergies commonly affect breathing
• Allergy medicines dehydrate the normally moist sinus passages

- Illness such as a cold or influenza also cause labored breathing
- Tissue scarring from surgery on the nasal passage
- General thickness of tissues found within the sinuses
- Nasal spray abuse agitates the sinuses and airway
- Snorting controlled substances
- Oversized tonsils and/or adenoids
- Goiter, a swollen thyroid gland
- Oversized tongue
- Obesity results in thickness of the neck and soft tissues
- Oversized stomach
- Consumption of alcohol
- Smoking
- Ageing

Some of these issues affect men more than women, like excessive girth of the stomach region. This is believed to part of the reason men in general experience more issue with snoring than women.

Also, controlled substances; prescribed, available over the counter, or illegal are associated with side effects that lead to snoring such as drying the sinuses and relaxing the tissues at the back of the throat and air passages.

We have looked over that snoring is and broken down the physical process. We have also gone over the many issues that can affect and cause snoring, so we must now look deeper in to the issue to discover the truly deleterious effect snoring can have on a person's wellbeing.

What is so Bad About Snoring?
The whole concept of snoring is somewhat subversive; this is where the largest danger with snoring lies,

how innocuous it is perceived by the majority of people. Snoring as word seems harmless enough, and this is a problem. The connotation of the word does not convey the true meaning of the action; when a person snores, their body is in a state where it is being deprived of oxygen and must therefore breathe much harder to force open the airway. Simply put snoring is a cry for help in the dark that says "I am not breathing!"

Because of this common perception of snoring, people become incredulous at the idea that snoring is a serious problem gives rise to health risks and emotional issues. This portion of the book addresses the severity of snoring and the many issues associated with it. Most people are ignorant to the fact that snoring, although common, is not normal, healthy or acceptable.

The Physical Aspects of Snoring
What needs to happen for people to understand what snoring truly represents is a change of perception; a dynamic shift of what snoring means. The gravity of the dangers of snoring cannot be stressed enough. What follows is an abridged list of physical health issues that are related to snoring.
• Sleep apnea
• Heart Disease
• Stroke
• Headaches
• Night sweats
• Heartburn
• Swollen limbs
• Weakened immune system
• Loss of hearing

Remember, this is only an abridged list; there are many more physical issues that are part of snoring. These issues are not exclusive to adults, and neither is snoring.

Snoring is encompasses all ages and genders making anyone susceptible to the many dangerous effects snoring can have. Let's take a closer look at one of the more serious issues related to snoring.

Sleep Apnea in Depth
Sleep Apnea is a silent killer that strikes in the dark when a person is at their most vulnerable; when a person is asleep. This alone should be enough to make anyone who snores, or even cares about a person who snores to seek out some resolution; find some way to provide relief when sleeping so as not to stop breathing altogether. The term apnea is taken from the ancient Greek use of the word meaning: absence of breathing. Sleep

Apnea is merely a precursor to asphyxiation.

The correlation between snoring and Sleep Apnea is direct: really snoring is just another word for Sleep Apnea. If snoring is caused by tissue blocking the air passage; this is an absence of breath. The sound associated with snoring if the vibration of the obstructive tissue is being vibrated by the body sensing this blockage and breathing with a sense of urgency. Sleep Apnea is when breathing stops; snoring is when the body forces itself to breath hard enough to open the blockage. The correlation is simple.

Sleep Apnea does not have to be fatal to have a negative effect on a person's health. Breathing provides the body with oxygen, it goes into the lungs and then into the bloodstream from where the oxygen it taken to all parts of the body. Sleep Apnea translates to not breathing; if we are not breathing, our body is starved of the oxygen it needs to survive and operate to its full capacity. A lack of oxygen causes an imbalance in the blood stream leading to an excess of carbon dioxide. Too much Carbon dioxide in the body creates a toxic state that can result in brain damage, heart disease or a stroke.

The Emotional Aspects of Snoring
Snoring does not affect the person who is actually snoring alone. Anyone close to a person who snores with any degree of severity understands this fact. How snoring affects the people around a person who snores is just as serious as the health risks involved. A person, who snores loudly; meaning as loud a running motorcycle or some other internal combustion device, can keep their partner from sleeping. A

loud snorer can disrupt the whole house through the course of the night, every night.

This should begin to expose the vast area of problems that can arise due to snoring. A person who sleeps with someone who snores, or maybe shares the same room, or shares a wall between rooms, even so far as to be in the same building knows that trying to get a full night of deep, restful sleep is an exercise in futility. There is a lot of frustration involved with situations like these because the person snoring may be unaware of it, or believe there is nothing that can be done for it. Snoring can come with a costly emotional price tag; the following are few examples of emotional disturbances resulting from snoring:
• Loss of sleep can cause depression or anxiety

- Break up of relationships, including marriages
- Eviction from dwelling for bothering tenants
- Clashing living partners or neighbors due to sleep disruption
- Poor performance at work leading to unemployment
- Short term and long term memory issues from lack of sleep
- Lack of compassion from those affected by snoring

These are but a few of the many emotional problems that are part and parcel of snoring. The effects of snoring are very far reaching and destructive to those subject to them.

Beneath the surface of each of these emotional states are the mental states associated to the person who snores and the person who has to deal with it.

A few of the emotional states caused from snoring follow:
• Exhaustion
• Frustration
• Resentment
• Anger
• Helplessness
• Anguish
• Desperation
• Low self esteem
• Confusion

It is not hard to see how lack sleep can affect ones demeanor, especially if it the loss of sleep is du to someone else's snoring. One can quickly lose empathy for a person who snores when they are the on being kept up. So how can the snoring issue be solved? There are different schools of thought and many approaches to alleviating snoring which will be discussed shortly, but first the surgical approach will be addressed and why it should not be the first choice.

Chapter Two: Snoring Surgery?

Living in the twenty first century affords wonderful advances in medicine and surgery. Snoring is something that has plagued mankind since time immemorial. A person who snores in this day and age does is lucky in the sense that the impact of snoring is really starting to be understood. Before taking any approach to stop snoring, take advantage of what the medical community has to offer; find out why you are snoring. Knowing the root cause behind a snore will help to point you in the right direction as to how to eliminate or mitigate the snore as much as possible. Available options for relief can include allergy medicine up to surgery, although surgery for snoring is rarely if ever the best choice.

Snoring Does Not Equal Surgery
Surgery is often the considered to be the ultimate remedy to many of life's problems. This does not always apply to snoring. In fact, the nature of surgery and snoring do not really go too well together. Surgery should be considered as the very last resort for several reasons. There are risks involved with any surgical process, and in many cases these risks are outweighed by the benefits; but this is usually the case where there are few if any other options to taking care of a problem that is affecting a person's health and well being.

Snoring Surgery
Surgery is an exploratory process. The very nature of what surgery is seems somewhat counterproductive to

solving something like snoring, especially when there are other methods to address the issue that are much less invasive and can be just as successful. Surgery causes scarring, and because it is an exploratory process, there is no way to know what a doctor is going to encounter until they are in the process of cutting and opening up the patient. Surgery can often be the actual cause of snoring after going through a procedure such as rhinoplasty.

The truth is that surgeries performed in an effort to resolve issues with snoring have not always yielded the desired result for a large percentage of people who have had it. Surgery for snoring is not a common process, and is not as reliable as some surgical procedures that are performed on a regular basis. Because snoring is the result of tissue blocking the air passage, the surgical answer is to remove any excess tissue that may be causing the blockage.

For certain people, this may be a reasonable and acceptable answer to their snoring problem, but this is most definitely not the case for the majority of people who snore.

Keep in mind that snoring is not always the source of the problem; snoring is more often, if not most often a symptom of something else in the body. The cause of an individuals snoring issue is going to be unique and distinct to each person, therefore, there is not one simple cure-all remedy to take care of every persons snoring problem. The following page contains an example of the complexity involved with snoring and how surgery does not always address the root cause.

An Example: From Snoring to Insurance

Let's look at something simple and non-medical: car insurance. Let's take 20 people who are considered bad drivers by their insurance companies. As a result of that dubious distinction, all of these drivers are going to face a premium increase of $500 when they're insurance is renewed.

Now, seen at a distance, it might appear as though all of these drivers are in the same boat (or same car, as it were). And given that assumption, a method to deal with this problem might be to simply give each of these people an extra $500 in cash. Really, as strange as that sounds, this is a way to solve this problem for each of these 20 drivers: they need to find $500 more to pay their insurance premium, and hence, that is what this so-called solution is going to do. Yet is this wise? No!

Some of those drivers – probably more than a few of them – are not going to actually correct why they might be classified as a "bad driver" by their insurance company. They simply won't know why they're bad drivers, and hence, some of them will likely remain a "bad driver", and face higher insurance premiums next year – but this time after a few more accidents or tickets.

As you can easily see, the real cause of the so-called "bad driving" isn't solved when each person is given a nice gift of $500 with which to pay his or her increased insurance premium. And since the problem isn't really solved, the bad driving can crop up again, and cause financial problems and even worse, it can endanger health and safety.

So when people readily turn to trachea tissue-cutting surgery to cure their snoring, they may quite easily be overlooking the real root cause of the snoring; something that may be related to diet, sleep position, jaw or tongue dysfunction, lifestyle, genetics, or be an indication of an even more serious health problem; an indication that could be dangerously suppressed (temporarily, at least), after a seemingly successful surgery.

Going to surgery as an easy, off-the cuff solution for snoring, is like giving these bad drivers $500 in cash. It may seem to solve their problem, but for many, it will just be a temporary fix; masking even deeper problems that can lead to severe consequences down the road, including Sleep Apnea.

Reasons to Deny Surgery for Snoring

Surgery is often prescribed as the first and only solution to a person who has a problem with snoring. Surgery in many cases, for different ailments, is considered as the first and only for of treatment there might be. This is not so with snoring. Where surgery can save lives and minimize suffering, it also comes with costs in addition to the finances involved. There are a multitude of reasons that surgery should not be considered due to the risks involved with surgery which include the following:

• Post operation cosmetic effects
• Infection
• Scare tissue and inflammation
• Costly follow-up surgical procedures
• Time intensive healing process
• Costly drugs to ease pain and manage swelling
• Potential of damage to speech and tone of voice

- Complications with swallowing
- Potential seepage from wound and hemorrhaging
- Potential for irritating dry mouth
- Potential for severe pain in ears

Overview of Surgical Procedures for Snoring

Surgery is a life saving tool that has saved countless lives, but in this day and age, there is a surgical procedure for just about everything. Some of these procedures can be frivolous and unnecessary. When it comes to snoring specifically, surgery is not a guaranteed solution to the problem. It is essential that anyone who deals with snoring, either directly or indirectly is aware of this when looking for a way to fix the problem.

The following examples go over the common surgical procedures for snoring and how they might disappoint the patient. These examples state the name of the surgical procedure, what it is designed to do and most importantly the many ill effects that have been reported as a result of each respective procedure.

The problems listed as a result of the different surgical processes are serious. These problems range from finances to long term or permanent issues the patient may have to deal with after undergoing snoring surgery. What each of these surgeries is actually designed to do can be an absolute turn off, and when you consider the problems associated with them, the compounded effects are something to be gravely considered when there are so many other options available. Again, this is why in most cases, surgery should be considered as a last resort, if at all.

These are the risks associated with surgical procedures for snoring specifically; there are other risks that are a part of any surgical procedure; but these other kinds of issues cannot be compared to the unique set of problems that snoring creates and the different surgeries designed to fix snoring. Cost for example, is always an issue, but should be taken into account for an issue like snoring whereas for an issue like cancer, or a failing organ, the cost must be incurred to preserve and improve life. Another risk is anesthesia. Being "put under" for surgery is not always the case, but for any kind of major surgery it is the case. Having surgery performed for snoring would require this and anesthesia has been known to result in complications if not death in some instances.

Tracheostomy
Create an opening in the trachea (sometimes this is called a tracheotomy)
- Irritating to tissues and possible scarring
- Requires follow-up surgery
- Nasal secretions can clog air pipe and lead to breathing difficulties

UPPP (Uvulopalatopharyngoplasty) expand the airway and end snoring
- Expensive
- May require follow-up surgery of obstruction occurs again
- Post-operation infection
- Possible speech defects
- Higher than normal
- Hemorrhage risk
- Swallowing problems
- Not effective for Sleep Apnea

LAUP (Laser Assisted Uvuloplasty)
Uses lasers to remove uvula and obstructing tissues, without removing tonsils or lateral tissues
- Dry mouth
- Changes to voice (to be avoided by people who require their voice to earn their living!)
- Pain in the ears
- Unpredictable success rate
- Can mask deeper problems and/or lead to new complications

CAPSO (Cautery-assisted palatal stiffening operation)
Burns the palate in order to stiffen it against vibration, and removes the mucosa along the uvula.
- Post-operation discomfort and pain
- Currently in experimental stages (unproven)
- Difficulty predicting if surgery will be successful and quite Expensive

Aside from these examples, there are other new kinds of snore specific surgeries that have been developed which include somnoplasty and snoreplasty. These procedures are new and as yet unproven to have any kind of reliable success rate in addition to not knowing what any long tem effects may arise from these kinds of surgeries for snoring.

In general surgery is a good thing, a very good thing; but this does not mean that surgery is the best step to take when looking to resolve an issue with snoring. To be clear; there are cases where surgery is absolutely the best possible solution for a person suffering from snoring and the positive effects resound just like the negative ones did when snoring was causing loss of sleep and all the negative health issues and frames of mind that go along with that.

Luckily there are other options available. Non-surgical answers to snoring abound, some of these remedies have been around for a long time, while others are relatively new. These less invasive steps to alleviating snoring are where the majority of relief from snoring comes from. Countless people use these alternative methods with great success around the world, making it easier for them and those around them to sleep and feel good which we will now take a look at.

Having already gone over the surgical aspects of snoring, the risks and procedures; we now turn our attention to the more common approaches to dealing with snoring. The non-surgical options for resolution of snoring can be broken down into different types of approaches: medicines, devices and appliances, changes in lifestyle concerning diet and exercise, sleeping habits and alternative forms of therapy for snoring. Any of these can be implemented with success depending on the root cause of the snoring, and knowing what that root cause is. This may require a combination approach, and will definitely require observation of the effects of these measures on the snoring issue itself in order to estimate how much relief results.

Medicinal Solutions

In many cases, prescribed medicines can provide a way out of the snoring nightmare. Drugs are prescribed to achieve relief from snoring by accomplishing these tasks:

• Unfurl the nasal airway
• Energize breathing
• Counteract deep R.E.M. sleep (Rapid Eye Movement)

R.E.M. sleep is an integral part of sleep. It is the deep state of sleep in which the body recoups vitality and allows the mind to stay sharp and healthy. The effect of these snore related drugs is to limit the depths to which the body can relax when in this state so as to keep the throat from relaxing too much and keeping the air passage open and free of obstruction thus leading to relief from snoring. Basically these medicines have the opposite effect of what happens when someone takes a sedative or has too much to drink. These things relax a person more than usual and can exacerbate an existing snoring problem, or cause a person who does not normally snore to do so.

There are over the counter drugs available from pharmacies intended specifically to clear nasal sinuses and air passages. These drugs are meant to treat cold or flu symptoms, but are also useful to snorers for the decongestive and antihistamine properties contained therein. Saline sprays, because they are sold in pharmacies as well are considered part of the same group. These sprays are not controlled substances, buy merely salt water used to keep sinuses and other tissues surrounding the air passages moist in an effort to reduce or eliminate vibration and thusly snoring.

Devices for Snoring

There are a number of devices out there to help people cope with their snoring. These items start with very basic items and go to the very complex. Most of these can be acquired at your local drugstore, on the internet and by catalogue. The most popular and effective anti-snore items follow.

The Sandler PillowTM

Named after the inventor of this type of pillow, this device is designed to eliminate snoring by obliging the sleeper to sleep on their side. This often promotes a closed mouth while sleeping and helps to minimize vibration and thereby cancels out any snoring.

The Snore Ball

Since its invention in the early 1900's this effective device has helped countless people to stop snoring by sleeping on their side. The snore ball is inserted in a pouch located on the back of a set of pajamas. When the sleeper goes to roll onto their back from sleeping on their side, the device makes this very uncomfortable, so the sleeper will resume the side sleeping position rather than sleeping on their back which is when most people snore. The snore ball can be any kind of ball that will create enough discomfort to keep one from sleeping on their back. Over time a habit is formed making the ball unnecessary.

Sleep Position Monitor

This electronic device basically accomplishes the same goal in a different manner. Instead of creating physical discomfort when a person lies on their back, which is when snoring occurs, the sleep position monitor starts to beep when the sleeper lies on their back. The beeping can be disturbing to others, but the point is that this device helps establish new sleeping behaviors. Anyone who has suffered a person snoring can deal with a little beeping until the problem is resolved. By learning a better way to sleep, the person will stop snoring and the beeping will not be an issue over time. Eventually the sleep position monitor may not be necessary either.

Nasal Strips
This is a simple yet highly effective device that has become popular for many people. The concept is basic, open up the nostrils to make breathing easier. The device consists of a springy plastic strip combined with and adhesive material. The strip is put on at bedtime and taken off in the

morning. The strips are so effective in maximizing breathing through the nose that they are used by many players of different sports. This is an over the counter remedy that anyone can use because there is absolutely no medicine involved. Even non snorers are using them to get better more restful sleep by breathing easier and recharging their body with more oxygen.

Nasal Dilators

Nasal dilators offer the same relief of opening up the nostrils to ease breathing, but take a slightly different approach than the nasal strips. This kind of device is actually a coil made of steel or plastic placed into the nostrils when going to sleep. The effect is easier breathing, less snoring.

Throat Sprays
This is another way to combat snoring. A simple spray to the back of the throat keeps the tissues well lubed in order to reduce or eliminate vibration. This is similar to a saline spray, the difference is what the spray consists of which in this case are specialized oils, not just salt water. Throat sprays are another form of simple, inexpensive, yet effective of combating snoring when used properly. Overuse of throat sprays can irritate the throat and then actually cause snoring. If an over the counter spray is not good enough, a doctor can prescribe a more effective version of the same implement.

Snore StopperTM
The snore stopper is a device that provides a negative association with snoring to make the person sleeping stop snoring. The device can be worn on the arm or the wrist and whenever

snoring is detected the device gives the sleeper a small jolt of electricity to get them to stop. Another version actually causes the tongue muscles to tense which opens the airway making it easier to breathe and hence stop snoring.

Snoring Appliances
Snoring appliances are applied inside the mouth to directly influence or affect the components of the mouth to eliminate snoring. These work to manipulate the tongue, jaw and palate in some combination to stop snoring and provide better rest.

Oral Appliances
These sets of tools are often designed by medical and dental professionals to help with the snoring dilemma. They have different names such as The EqualizerTM and The SilencerTM. By influencing the parts of the mouth

these devices affect three basic properties to eliminate snoring; they are:
• Keeping the mouth closed so that a person may not snore by making the trachea vibrate.
• Positioning the jaw in a forward placement to keep the tongue from sliding back and blocking the airway.
• Opening the airway as much as possible to ease breathing and prevent snoring.

Tongue Retaining Appliances
This style of appliance specifically targets the tongue. The effect of this appliance keeps the tongue forward by using suction to train the tongue not to lay back over the airway. This increases airflow making it easier to breathe and preventing the vibration that causes snoring. A tongue retainer is for people who cannot or will not sleep on their side, and although a

tongue retainer may be less than comfortable, it is a highly effective option.

Mandibular Advancement Appliances

Shortened to MAA, this is a splint style of appliance that are basically like a mouth guard used in sports. This keeps the jaw locked in a position that keeps it from moving back and creating an obstruction that leads to snoring. These must be custom molded by a dental professional and may be somewhat costly but are a great way to stop snoring.

Thronton Adjustable Positioners

The SilencerTM is a popular example of this kind of device, which was created by Dr. Thronton in the 1990's. This is an expensive option, but for a reason; it is adjustable and is sometimes crafted from titanium. These are often referred to as TAPs, and are similar in nature to MAAs in that they move the jaw forward in order to keep the airway open and prevent snoring.

Palate Lifters

Also known as lip shields, or lip lifters, this appliance augments the palate to keep from vibrating and causing a person to snore. This is an option to consider, although there has yet to be a resolute opinion in the efficiency of this type of appliance.

Continuous Positive Airway Pressure

This appliance is designed to tackle Sleep Apnea specifically. It works similar to an oxygen mask. The mask is worn on the face, or over the nose and keeps what is called positive pressure in the airway which prevents the collapse of tissue and eases breathing to the point of controlling ones blood pressure while asleep.

Allergies

Allergies have been linked to snoring, but because there are so many allergens, and each person is different, it is up to the individual to observe when they are snoring and what they are allergic to. Any kind of allergic reaction can lead to snoring, so when you are suffering from allergies, whether they a food allergies or pet, you need to take notice and take the appropriate measures to handle these allergies.

Weight

If you are overweight and snore, you can bet that your snoring is at least in part related to your obesity. Losing weight has a wide variety of health benefits, including better sleep by not snoring. This has to do with your diet and eating habits, so if you shape up, you may stop snoring altogether.

Eating Habits

Certain foods cause congestion, like dairy, fried foods, junk food and sweets. If you snore, your diet probably has something to do with it. Eating a healthier diet can improve your health as well as minimize if not alleviate any snoring. There are foods that are considered to be beneficial for people who snore, which consist mostly of leafy greens.

Clean Living

Your habits can determine whether or not you will snore. Healthy habits actually prevent snoring. Drinking and sleeping pills are known to cause snoring; use these in moderation. If you smoke and you snore, chances are quitting will help you sleep better by not snoring. Caffeine has been linked to respiratory issues, so keep your intake to a minimum.

Lifestyles and Snoring – Exercise

Exercise in general is good for the body, and helps to achieve more restful sleep. Healthy habits help prevent to minimize snoring, but there are snoring specific exercises one can do.

Throat Work Out

Toning the muscles of the throat can really improve the breathing process when sleeping, thus helping with snoring if not eradicating it all together. There are a few options to stress the muscles systems that affect snoring. You can firmly hold a pencil between your teeth for up to five minutes. Pressing a finger to the chin with moderate pressure for a few minutes builds jaw strength. Also holding the tip of the tongue firmly against the bottom front teeth strengthens the tongue. These are exercises that can be done anytime, anywhere. These should not be painful, and the more these exercises are implemented, the better the results will be.

Sleep Factors
One needs to consider the way in which one sleeps and how that affects the way you breathe at night. Sleeping on your back promotes snoring, but having a good pillow, or sleeping with something under the chin can help to stop snoring. Anything to keep the mouth shut during sleep is a big help. Your sleep environment plays a role in snoring too. A humidifier will help keep the throat and sinuses moist, and making the room as dark and quiet as possible helps to reduce stress, and

calm the person sleeping to the point that breathing becomes easier.

Snoring Therapy Alternatives
Here are some other approaches one can try when dealing with snoring; these have been around for some time because of how successful they have been in combating snoring. A warm drink before bed; herbal tea can really help alleviate snoring. Relaxation techniques to calm the mind and practice breathing techniques like Tai Chi and Yoga have been of great benefit to many snorers.

Other forms of relaxation include meditation and massage, or even just soothing music. Homeopathic medicines offer many ways to deal with snoring too. These include products like Snore StopTM and Y-SnoreTM. Homeopathic alternatives look to achieve the same end result in different ways, such as dissolving blockages in the nose and throat or lubrication with natural products. Magnetic therapy is popular in china and can help ameliorate snoring by affecting the nerves found in the nose. Magnets can be put all over the body to achieve results that improve issues with snoring. This applies even to weight loss which can in turn affect snoring. Even hypnosis has been used to help control snoring by some, although many are skeptical of this practice as it is not a recognized successful solution to snoring.

Other more "alternative" therapies are based on light and color, or in other circumstances gems and crystals as sources of healing power. These latter examples have yet to be established as effective by science or medicine, but the power of belief can be enough to produce the placebo effect. So as long as the end result is the cessation of snoring, any means can be tried and tested to see if they work for a given individual.

Conclusion

I hope you'll have found your solution to get rid of snoring!

If therapy or changing your habits isn't helping you getting rid of snoring surgery can be an effective way to solve your sleep apnea disorder. Please consult a physician for his or her opinion about the best procedure.

Will you review this book?

Reviewing this book will ensure potential readers know what to expect out of buying this (e-)book. It would be great if you are willing to share your experience!

www.ingramcontent.com/pod-product-compliance
Lightning Source LLC
Chambersburg PA
CBHW071000180526
45168CB00003B/1221